MOVE THE FAT

20 Easy and Effective Exercises to Fight Obesity for Beginners, Seniors, Men, and Women

VINH NGUYEN

CONTENTS

INTRODUCTION

Weight loss is one of the most popular goals in the world for a good reason. Being obese or overweight can be the source of many problems. Obesity was linked to 4.7 million deaths in 2017, representing 8% of the total deaths for the year.

As a leading cause of premature and preventable deaths, obesity is a central theme in various ailments like diabetes, hypertension, cardiovascular diseases, stroke, infertility, premenstrual syndrome, hormonal imbalance, certain cancers, and chronic inflammation. Apart from health conditions, obesity can affect self-esteem and confidence and lead to personality issues. Obesity is a worldwide pandemic, and the statistics make for grim reading:

- *About 13% of the world's population is obese.*

- *Statistics from the CDC (Centers for Disease Control and Prevention) suggest that 42% of adult Americans are obese.*

- *The percentage of children aged 5 to 19 who are overweight or obese has risen from 4% in 1975 to around 16%.*

- *Obesity is responsible for $147 billion in medical costs annually in the U.S.*

Unfortunately, most weight loss goals, especially for obese people, are not met. This is not a big surprise since weight loss plans usually involve regular exercise, and most people cannot make a consistent habit. So, losing extra weight seems to be an impossible task for many people. Therefore, I have written this book to help you gain the upper hand in your quest to get fit and healthy.

Obesity simply occurs when the rate of calories consumed is significantly larger than the calories expended as energy over a long period. If the amount of food you continue to consume exceeds the energy you burn, the extra calories will be stored by your body and make you obese. To fix this, you can either attempt to reduce the amount of food you eat or increase your energy expenditure.

That is why diets and exercise are the only two ways to lose weight. However, diets are notoriously hard to stick to, can be time- and effort-demanding, and there is no guarantee they will work. The effect of exercises, on the other hand, are relatively predictable.

Are you obese and need an exercise program to lose the extra pounds? Do you want to know the best exercises for your body type? Are you tired of the pains and aches that come with obesity? Do you want the right knowledge and tips for common exercises? This book will provide answers to these and many more questions.

I admit that exercising can be challenging for obese people. It is harder to complete reps and stick to the plan. For this reason, you must choose the right exercises and carry them out correctly. I will spell out twenty of the best choices you can make in this book and provide some guidance on how to do them correctly. Depending on their effect, these exercises will be divided into three groups (chapters).

Before we dive in, I should mention that losing weight is not just about burning calories. It is about creating a calorie deficit. For this to happen, you need to burn calories (exercise) and reduce the number of calories you eat (dieting). I am suggesting that exercising alone is not enough. You also have to adopt a healthy diet to get the best result.

But that is not all. There are two ways in which exercise causes weight loss. Number one: they make you burn calories during the workout. Number two: they increase your rate of metabolism so that you continue to burn calories long after the workout. The technical name for this is the afterburn effect, and it can last for up to 24 hours.

I am telling you this because I may recommend some exercises that are not very good at burning calories directly. This is especially true for strength training and endurance exercises. However, they have an excellent afterburn effect. They also improve muscle mass, thus increasing the body's ability to burn fat by over 2½ times more.

One advantage of choosing different exercises is that you can combine and mix them to a significant effect. As a result, you burn more calories during and after the workout. You also get to train and strengthen a larger range of muscle groups. Finally, tired muscle groups get more time to rest, rebuild, and recover before you give them another workout. Recovery is crucial for both weight loss and muscle building.

With that out of the way, let's get the ball rolling.

Good luck!

CHAPTER 1

CARDIO EXERCISES

Cardiovascular exercises, also known as aerobics, are the best for losing weight. Some can burn up to 10 to 12 calories per minute, although that depends on the intensity of the exercise and your body fat ratio.

Apart from burning fat, cardio exercises have other benefits. They can also improve stress levels, blood circulation, lung health, heart health, muscle strength, and endurance. Every muscle group in the body benefits from cardio, and the extent of the benefits depends on the exercise's intensity.

There are two types of cardio exercises: high intensity and low intensity. As the name suggests, the former raises your heart rate much higher and thus causes more calorie loss. They are also more demanding to perform. Examples are burpees, dancing, running, mountain cycling, and intense cycling or swimming. On the other hand, examples of low-intensity cardio exercises are walking, jogging, and almost every activity mentioned in the other category in a less intense form.

The American Heart Association says the average individual should put in around 75 minutes of high-intensity or 150 minutes of moderate-intensity cardio per week for a healthy life. I recommend splitting that into five sessions a week. However, for the best results for weight loss or any other fitness goal, you have to combine high-intensity cardio with low-intensity cardio like in high-intensity interval training (HIIT) and cardio with strength training.

1. Walking

Walking is not the first exercise that comes to mind when looking to lose weight. Nevertheless, it is the one I choose to start with for a few reasons. It doesn't cost much money or effort. Yet, studies show it can help burn between 3.5 to 5.2 calories per minute. You can only enjoy maximum benefits by engaging in it regularly. But the fact remains that even a low-intensity exercise like this can do a lot.

So, if you are interested, I suggest 20- to 30-minute walks 2 or 3 times every week. If you can't find the time, how about leaving the car behind on your trips to the grocery store or walking the dog? You can make things more challenging and probably burn more calories by walking briskly or uphill or wearing weighted vests.

2. Swimming

Like walking and its higher intensity counterparts, jogging and running, swimming also exercises all of the body's muscle groups. The biggest difference is that swimming is less harsh on the joints. And because of this, it is more appropriate for anyone with knee issues.

Still, swimming can help you burn up to 8 calories per minute. However, that depends on the intensity of the exercise. The most intense swimming styles that burn the most calories are butterfly stroke, breaststroke, and backstroke. Most likely, you will be

7

combining multiple styles within a session.

I suggest three to five sessions every week to use swimming for weight loss. Start small and try to avoid eating before entering the pool. You can increase session lengths gradually and even add water weights or swimming routines as you improve.

3. Burpees

Burpees are one of those exercises that you will find on almost every exercise regimen for weight loss, and for a good reason, too. It is a compounding exercise that is great for building muscle mass and burning calories. It burns about ten calories per minute. So, burpees are almost the perfect exercise for weight loss. The only potential problem is they can be very physically demanding. Still, I recommend them even if you can only last for a few reps. That will still do some good.

You can also do it as part of HIIT sessions. It means combining a short burst of intense exercise with periods of low intensity. Here is an example: one minute of burpees with two minutes of jogging. This gives your body recovery breaks and allows you to last longer while also utilizing the higher fat-burning attributes of intense physical exercises.

Variations of burpees include push-ups, one-handed, sumo squats, broad jump burpees, star jump burpees, and side burpees. Here is how to do a simple burpee:

1. *Stand with your feet at shoulder width*
2. *Squat and lay your palms on the floor in front of you*
3. *Jump into the high plank position*
4. *Jump back into position 2*
5. *Return to position 1*
6. *Repeat 8 to 10 times per set*

You can start as slowly as needed. But pace equals intensity which equals more fat loss.

4.   Cycling

Like all cardio, cycling is an excellent exercise for fighting obesity. It doesn't matter if it's an actual or stationary bike or whether you are riding on rough or smooth terrain, you can still burn lots of calories. Studies say cycling burns around ten calories per minute. The best part is that it doesn't put too much strain on your knees and joints compared to running. However, mountain biking can be quite physically demanding and requires more skill.

So, it is all about deciding how hard you can push your body to make it sweat while also limiting the risks of injury. Of course, stationary cycling is the safest, so you may want to start with that. But I suggest getting an actual bike to enjoy the outdoors. I recommend two to three sessions per week. You can even adopt it as your secondary means of transportation for running errands or going to work.

5. Jogging/Running

Running is, without doubt, the most common exercise of all time. And that is a testament to both its many benefits and how easy it is to get started. Those benefits include everything that I mentioned when discussing cardio. But the main reason for its appearance on this list is the ability to burn a whopping 9 to 15 calories per minute. Of course, this depends on factors like intensity and muscle mass, but the fact remains that no other exercise can compare to this one. The only problem is the strain that it puts on your joints.

If you want to use running for weight loss, I recommend three to seven sessions per week. You can do it any time of the day, but I recommend morning or evening. In the morning, jogging or running prepares your body and mind for the day ahead. In the evening, they offer a way to relax and relieve stress. My other suggestions include:

- *A warm-up before each session (Stretching and even slow jogging will do.)*
- *Dress for the occasion (It doesn't matter if you are running outdoors or using a treadmill, you still need the right clothes and shoes.)*
- *Use HIITs (Combine jogging and running for HIITs. Try a 45-second burst, followed by a 75-second jog.)*

6. Dancing

Surprised? Yes, dancing can qualify as an exercise and is efficient at losing weight. It can burn up to 13 calories per minute. The best part is that you don't have to learn any special moves. That means you can be burning calories, dancing alone in your room, or on a day out with friends. Just put on your favorite song and move your body.

However, this approach won't be enough if you want to rely on dancing alone as a weight-loss strategy. You need structured and consistent sessions with dance moves that require shaking and, by default, exercising every part of your body. So, I recommend taking a hip hop, Zumba, freestyle, ballet, or ballroom dancing class.

The only potential problem is that some of these classes may be too demanding. But as always, the goal is to get started and increase the challenge gradually. Doing a little bit is better than doing nothing. Plus, the guidance and companionships in real-life dancing classes will help.

7.   Step hop

Here is another cardio exercise that can help you lose fat at a rate of 7 calories per minute. You also enjoy all the other benefits of cardio exercises. Step hop focuses mainly on the lower body, especially the legs. Its effects improve overall balance, endurance, and mobility.

I also recommend it because it is beginner-friendly and gentle on the knees. For weight loss, I recommend the basic version (which I will teach below) and the squat pop over, stepping match, and side stepper variations.

1.   *Stand upright with your feet slightly apart*

2.   *Keep your arms by your sides*

3.   *Take a step forward*

4.   *Hop and raise the lead leg and the opposite arm*
simultaneously

5.   *Step back and repeat for the other leg and arm*

Bend the raised leg at the knee and raise it until the knee reaches hip level. Next, bend the raised arm at the elbow and raise it until the elbow reaches shoulder level.

CHAPTER 2

WEIGHT-TRAINING OR MUSCLE BUILDING EXERCISES

The exercises in this category focus on specific muscle groups and confer strength on them. Nevertheless, they are an excellent option for weight loss due to the afterburn effect they produce. Also, you can customize them to target specific parts of the body to address weaknesses. For instance, they can be used to improve lower back pain issues.

8. Lunges

Over the last few years, lunges have become a popular exercise among those looking to tighten and enlarge their glutes. However, its benefits are beyond that. Lunges strengthen the entire lower body, leading to better posture, stamina, fitness, and athleticism.

Remember that I said the best exercises for weight loss exercise a wide variety of muscle groups? Well, lunges don't fit in that category. However, it builds muscle mass. I hope you remember that this will increase the rate of metabolism, which means a faster rate of calorie and fat loss. You can still lose up to 5 calories per minute while engaging in lunges alone. But you will get the better effects by combining it with cardio exercises.

Common variations of lunges that can help fight obesity are forward, lateral, reverse, walking, jump, side, and diagonal lunges. Here is a quick guide on how to perform a basic lunge:

1. *Stand upright, with heels planted on the ground and palms on both sides of your waist*

2. *Take a step forward with one leg while bending the other at the knee*

3. *Plant the front leg on its heel (Keep your back*

straight while doing this, don't lean. If done right, the knee of the back leg will be closer to the floor.)

4. *Return to the starting position*

5. *Repeat for movement for the second leg*

6. *Repeat multiple times for both legs*

7. *Do 8 to 10 repetitions per set*

It is crucial to get the form right for this exercise, as mistakes can lead to injury. Also, you have to understand that it puts lots of strain on the knees. The front knee for each repetition carries the bulk of the entire body weight. So, you may want to avoid lunges if you have knee issues. It also doesn't hurt to wear knee braces even if your knees are perfect.

Once again, start small and scale up gradually. For example, increase the number of sets and add free weights to make things more challenging.

9. Sit-ups

The sit-up has always been a staple of most workout routines. One reason for this is that it is beginner-friendly and doesn't need equipment. When done right, it works a large group of muscles, including the rectus abdominis, obliques, and transverse abdominis. There is also a contraction of the hip and neck flexors as you perform sit-ups. In addition, sit-ups can help you with abs definition, strengthening the core.

Even though it is a strength-building exercise, sit-ups can still help you burn up to 5 to 9 calories per minute, depending on the intensity. However, it is essential to state that sit-ups come with an increased risk of injuries compared to its cousin, the crunch. The major difference between these two exercises is that sit-ups have a longer range of motion and have fewer variations. Here is how to do a basic sit-up:

1.   *Lie down on your back with your knees bent*

2.   *Cross your palms under your head and relax your body*

3.   *Using your core muscles, lift your upper body towards your knees and exhale*

4.   *Slowly return to your starting position*

You can do any number of sets you are comfortable with for now and scale up later. It can be divided into multiple sessions spread throughout the day. However, you don't have to worry about that for now. Grow at your own pace!

10. Squats

Squatting is another exercise that has recently become

popular with those looking to build their gluteal region. Like lunges, it also works the lower body. But that is not all. The lower parts of the upper body also benefit. Squats exercise and strengthen the muscles of the calves, glutes, hamstrings, abdomen, and lower back.

Eventually, those body parts will become stronger. Posture and athleticism also improve. And as for weight loss, it can help you burn up to 5 calories per minute. Now, this varies depending on the intensity and variation. The best squat variations for losing weight are loaded ones like the goblet or front squat. You may also like the box squat, banded squat, sumo squat, heel elevated squat, and back squat.

How to do a weighted front squat (using a barbell bar):

1.   *Stand with your feet at shoulder width*

2.   *Hold a bar in both hands*

3.   *Bend your elbows to lift the bar until it's in front of your chest*

4.   *Bend your knees to squat*

5.   *Return to the starting position*

6.   *Repeat 6 times per set*

11. Dumbbell rolls

Free weights like barbells, kettlebells, and dumbbells are crucial when building up your arsenal of exercise equipment because you can use them to spice up almost any exercise. So, get them even if you don't plan to try this particular exercise. But I bet you will because it is beginner-friendly and can help you lose about three calories per minute. Plus, it is one of those exercises that work an extensive range of muscle groups.

However, the primary beneficiaries of the dumbbell roll are your back, arms, shoulders, and core. As a result, your endurance, athletics, posture, balance, and grip improve while your back strengthens. This exercise has several variations, such as the one-arm dumbbell roll and the inclined bench dumbbell roll. Here is how to do the basic one:

1.   *Hold a dumbbell in each hand*

2.   *Stand with your legs at shoulder width and arms by your side*

3.   *Bend your hips to shift your upper body forward (Try to form a 45-degree angle between your upper and lower body)*

4.   *Your knees can bend slightly, but don't let your feet leave the ground*

5.   *Bend your right elbow to raise the dumbbell on that hand to your hips*

6. *Reverse the last action*

7. *Repeat 5 and 6 times for the left hand*

8. *Repeat 5 to 7 or 8 to 12 times per set*

12. Single-leg deadlifts

The single-leg deadlift exercises the muscles of the glute, ankles, core, and hamstrings. It is one of those referred to as "compounding exercises." This means that it exercises a larger than average range of muscle groups. In this case, it is both the lower and upper body. As a result, balance, mobility, endurance, and posture improve. Those benefits (being able to burn calories and its beginner-friendliness) are my reasons for adding the single-leg deadlift to this list.

You have to scale up the intensity and length of your sessions to get the best out of this exercise. Sometimes, this could mean trying different variations. So, apart from the basic version, I recommend integrating kettlebell and barbell techniques.

1. *Stand with your legs at shoulder width and knees slightly bent*

2. *Shift your weight to your right leg*

3. *Drive the left leg straight back while hinging your upper body forward simultaneously (It is like*

taking a bow with one leg extended backward.)

4. *Return to the starting position*

5. *Repeat for the second leg*

6. *Repeat the exercise 5 to 8 times per set*

I recommend doing single-leg deadlifts 3 to 4 times a week. You can take a minute rest between sets. Then up the ante by reducing rest time, adding weight, and increasing the number of reps later down the line.

13. Planks

The plank doesn't involve a lot of physical movement and thus has limited ability to burn calories. But if you get the form right, it contracts the affected muscles in a way that burns 2 to 5 calories per minute. The directly affected muscles are in the lower back, hips, glutes, abdominal area, arms, legs, and pelvis. As a result, the muscles become leaner (having lost fat), and posture improves.

Some plank variations are walking, side, reverse, and leg-raise plank. Here is how to do the basic version:

1. *Lie face down, using your forearms and toes as support*

2. *Keep your feet slightly apart and your elbows at shoulder width*

3.   Engage your core, tighten your glutes, and make your body into a straight line

4.   Hold for at least a minute

It is more important to get the form right than hold it for longer. Still, try to hold the pose for longer as you get better at it.

14. Glute bridge

The glute bridge is another low-intensity strength-training exercise that you will love. It is easy to perform, yet burns up to 7 calories per minute. It does this by working the muscles of the hamstrings and glutes, ultimately resulting in better posture and stamina. I recommend trying the single-leg bridge, elected feet, and straightened-leg variations for a beginner to lose weight. Start with this version. You will need a mat, but any comfortable surface should work.

1.   Lie on your back with your hands by your side

2.   Raise your knees to plant your feet below them, close to your buttocks

3.   Squeeze the muscles of your buttocks and abdomen, then lift your hips to near the same height as your knees (You don't have to raise it too high until it snaps.)

4.   *Engage your core and hold the position for between 20 and 30 seconds.*

5.   *Return to number 2 and repeat step 3 to 4*

6.   *Do 8 reps per set*

15. Crunches

Crunches are like cousins to sit-ups and toe touches. The abdominal muscles receive a lot of attention. Once again, I don't want you to assume that this means it helps burn belly fat. Instead, focus on how it tones muscles, strengthens the core, and burns about 4 to 5 calories per minute. It may not seem like much, but you are getting an exercise that is perfect for beginners. Plus, you can improve the results by combining it with cardio exercises. So, here is how to do crunches:

1.   *Lie on your back*

2.   *Bend your knees to lift them and plant the soles of your feet on the ground*

3.   *Keep your leg at shoulder length*

4.   *Cross your palms at the back of your head*

5.   *Engage your core and lift your upper body*

6.   *Lower your upper body back to the floor*

7.   *Repeat step 5 and 6 for 15 to 20 times per set*

16. Farmers' walk

A farmers' walk aims to build and strengthen muscles in the glutes, triceps, and biceps. I am not implying it won't help you burn calories. Farmers' walk is more commonly found in strong men's activities. (Don't worry! We will be using much lighter weights.) You can use dumbbells, kettlebells, and an empty trap bar or barbell bar. Here is a dumbbell variation:

1. *Select two dumbbells of the same weight*

2. *Stand upright with your feet at shoulder width and a dumbbell on each side*

3. *Bend at the knees and hips to pick up one dumbbell in each hand*

4. *Return to the standing position*

5. *Take 15 to 30 steps forward*

6. *Bend at the knees and hips to set down the dumbbells*

7. *Return to the standing position*

8. *Take a rest*

9. *Repeat*

Don't worry about speed. Instead, focus on gradually increasing the weight size, the number of steps, and sessions.

24

17. Push-ups

Push-ups are perhaps the most common bodyweight exercise in the world today. They are easy to do and very effective at strengthening the core, the upper body, and the lower back and kickstarting the afterburn effect. You can also add many modifications to your routine to suit your purpose.

The primary targets of push-ups are the pectorals, triceps, and deltoid muscles. However, because you have to pull your core inwards towards your spine, they also increase the abdomen and lower back strength.

The classic push-up form is well known, but it is difficult to repeat over a short period, especially if you are already obese or not used to the exercise. I advise people to aim for at least three sets of 12 reps each, but many people cannot sustain that. If you are one of them, you can start with even ten push-ups daily. Then, slowly increase this figure each time you find it easy to complete. Many people complete 300 to 500 sets daily.

Here is how to do the classic push-ups:

1.   *Lie face down on all fours (your palms and toes) and keep your back flat in the plank position (Your*

25

hand should be held at shoulder width with the fingers turned inwards.)

2. *Slowly lower yourself until your chin or chest is almost touching the ground (Your elbows may flare out until they attain a 90 degrees position.)*

3. *Then, slowly press on the ground with your hands and raise your entire body upwards until your arms are fully extended at the elbow and you are in the plank position again*

4. *Keep your spine, back, and head straight through the whole process*

5. *One downward and upward movement constitutes one rep*

Try the bent-knee push-up or the incline push-up if you find the classic push-up too hard. You can make the routine more challenging by trying a decline push-up where your leg is raised above the rest of the body. The clapping push-up and diamond push-up are other harder variants.

CHAPTER 3

EXERCISES THAT IMPROVE FLEXIBILITY

Flexibility exercises increase your range of movement, prevent injuries, and improve recovery time. They are also suitable for warming up for more intense exercises and can make a huge difference. You can also combine them easily with some of the exercises from the other groups.

18. Pilates

If you are surprised to find Pilates on this list, you will

also have the same reaction after realizing that my next recommendation is yoga. There is no denying that neither of these leaps to mind when you think of weight loss.

The biggest effect they have on the body is to improve flexibility, core strength, balance, and posture. For that to happen, the entire body has to become leaner, which means less fat and more muscles. As said earlier, this increases metabolism. So, both Pilates and yoga help to lose fat. For Pilates, the rate is around 2.8 to 4 calories burnt per minute.

However, that is not the only way Pilates can lead to weight loss. Its effect on the mind (improving mindfulness and discipline) also makes it easier to stick to your workout routine and avoid unhealthy eating habits or other unhelpful habits that can impair your weight loss goal. So, in the end, both the physical and mental benefits of Pilates create a compounding effect.

The best types of Pilates for dealing with obesity are those that prioritize movement and total body workout. Good examples are plank jacks, V-ups, swan poses, and roll-up poses. I suggest three 50-minute or seven 15-minute sessions per week.

19. Yoga

Everything I said about Pilates also applies to yoga. That includes the mental and physical benefits and the compounding effects. Even the tips for using Pilates for weight loss (three 50-minute or seven 15-minute sessions per week) also apply. The only major differences are the number of calories burnt per minute and the techniques. So, let's discuss them.

Yoga burns about 3 to 5.6 calories per minute. The best techniques for weight loss are plank pose, warrior pose, triangle pose, downward dog, and power yoga. As with Pilates, these are techniques that prioritize full-body workouts. You can combine them at will. As always, start simple and raise the duration gradually.

20. Toe touches

Everyone sees toe touches as an abs exercise, but it has other benefits like improving balance, posture, and mobility. And here is the funny part: it is not even that great for toning abs. It will, however, make you lose five calories per minute. So, this exercise is an excellent addition to any weight loss routine.

However, it is essential to get the form right because it relies on muscle contortion over physical movement. So, follow these directions carefully:

1. *Lie on your back, with your body straightened and arms resting by your sides*

2. *Lift your legs as high as possible without lifting your lower back or being too uncomfortable (It's okay if your knees bend slightly.)*

3. *Lift your upper body and stretch forth your hands to touch each foot (Don't worry if you can't touch them.)*

4. *Return to the starting position and repeat*

5. *Do 10 to 15 reps per set*

Engage your core and abdomen to raise and lower your upper body instead of using the momentum of your arms. You need to keep the movements slow and deliberate. You can also inhale and exhale to mark the beginning and end of each rep.

CONCLUSION

Thank you for reading this book. I am very certain you have learned new exercises that can make a difference. I am also sure you have learned new tips about the exercises you already knew.

Exercises are a must in the battle against obesity. However, every effective fitness plan has to be built on the right choices of exercises in the right routine. I have attempted to simplify the process of choosing the right exercises for you. You can now choose between the three categories of exercises discussed in this book to create a calorie-burning factory out of your body.

I must also remind you that it is vital for you to eat

right and rest adequately to see faster results. It is now time for you to write an action plan for getting back into shape. Do not just expect things to happen to you randomly. Create the right conditions.

Choose the right time to exercise, build a support system, and deploy consistency to see the changes you have always wanted. Obesity is a killer, but it becomes powerless the more you move your body around. Weight loss may be hard to achieve, but it can become a fun-filled, rewarding journey to optimal health with the right exercises.

Good luck!

ABOUT THE AUTHOR

Vinh Nguyen sees himself as the "happiest author on earth." His life goal is to help as many people as possible to learn to be happy. One book at a time. He believes that you can be happy if you choose to exercise the power you already have within yourself.

Vinh was born and bred in Vietnam and lives (happily ever after) in New Zealand.

BY THE SAME AUTHOR

- 10 Proven Ways to Relieve Stress Now: An Essential Hack for a Better Life
- How to Sleep Faster Better Smarter Naturally: An Essential Easy Guide for Your Best Life
- Start Your Exercise Routine and Keep the Motivation Forever: A Simple Guide for Your Life Fitness
- Meditate for Life: A Simple Guide to Start Your Daily Meditation Journey and Love It Forever
- Muscle Building for Men After 40: A Life Changing Strength Training Guide for the Best Body In Your 40s and Beyond
- Lost It at 30: A Simple Weight Loss Guide for Women in their 30s, 40s, and Beyond

Printed in Great Britain
by Amazon